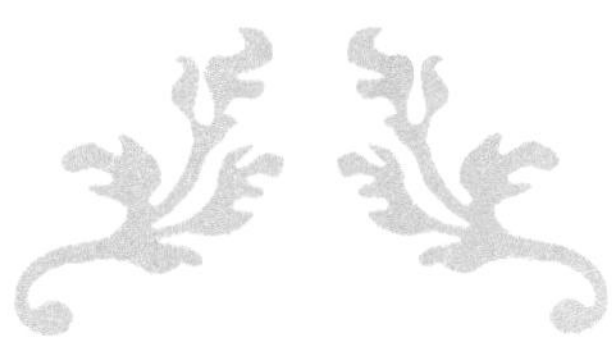

MEDITERRANEAN DIET COOKBOOK FOR SENIORS 2024

Complete Guide to Mediterranean Cooking for Older Men & Women with Easy Delicious Recipes, Food Chart, and 28-Day Meal Plan to Improve Health and Vitality

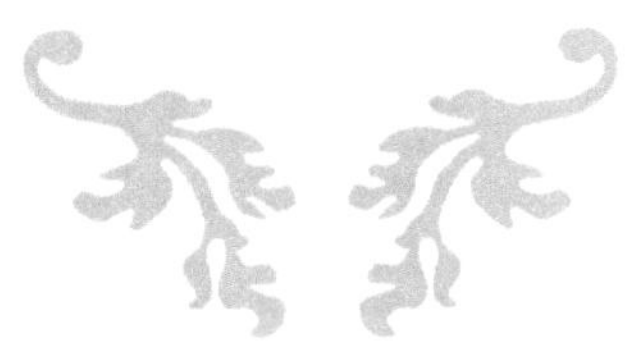

DR. ANGELA COOK

Also by Dr. Angela Cook

Scan the QR code to access other books by Dr. Angela Cook.

Mediterranean Diet Cookbook for Seniors 2024

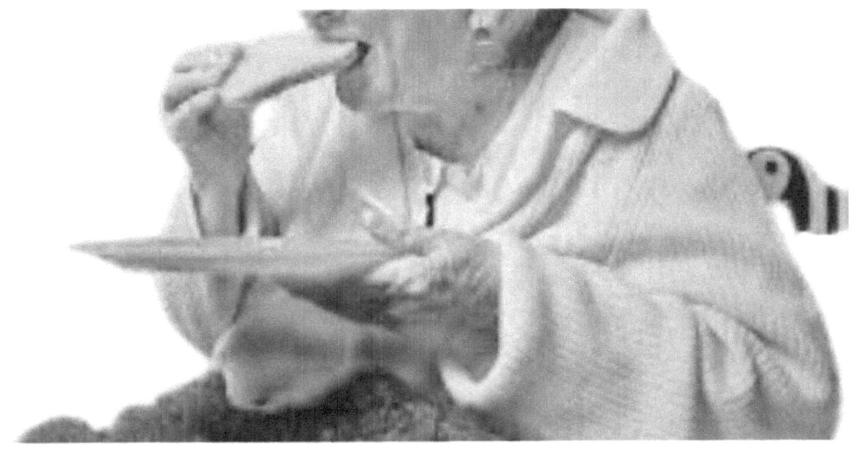

Complete Guide to Mediterranean Cooking for Older Men &
Women with Easy Delicious Recipes, Food Chart, and 28-Day Meal
Plan to Improve Health and Vitality

Dr. Angela Cook

TABLE OF CONTENTS

Dedication

This book is dedicated to all the vivacious and knowledgeable seniors who are adopting the Mediterranean way of life. You are the free spirits who know the true meaning of tasting life's delicacies. We are all inspired by your path toward greater health and energy through a Mediterranean diet. May the gastronomic explorations you undertake offer happiness, sustenance, and innumerable precious moments spent with loved ones. May this cookbook be a devoted ally on your journey towards well-being. Cheers to your good health, joy, and a lifelong love of life that only gets better with age.

With sincere commitment,

Dr. Angela Cook

About the Author

With a great deal of expertise in helping elders achieve better health, Dr. Angel Cook has a deep commitment to their well-being. She has demonstrated exceptional empathy and a thorough comprehension of the various difficulties elders encounter while navigating the intricacies of aging throughout her career. Her contacts with people like Sarah, Robert, and Maria have demonstrated her capacity to build solid, dependable connections with her senior clients, encouraging communication and cooperation.

Dr. Cook's approach is intrinsically personalized, acknowledging the distinct requirements and inclinations of every senior. This is demonstrated in her work with James, who was able to accomplish notable weight reduction and improved mobility with her customized coaching. Her technique is based on personalization, which guarantees that her recommendations correspond with each person's unique health status and nutritional needs, resulting in more favorable outcomes.

Dr. Cook's advocacy work for education has been a defining feature of her career. She has continuously shown that she is dedicated to educating seniors about the Mediterranean diet and its possible benefits, providing them with important information that enables them to make decisions about their health that are well-informed.

Seniors like Mary, who have been able to control their blood pressure better thanks to their increased understanding of diet, have found resonance with this educational position.

One common subject in Dr. Cook's conversations with senior citizens is celebration. Her journey has been interspersed with times of celebration, whether it be for the accomplishments of people like Patricia, who have embraced the Mediterranean diet with hope and zeal, or for the more subdued but no less meaningful successes of others. These victories demonstrate that achieving greater health is a realistic objective and demonstrate Dr. Cook's commitment to assisting seniors in living fulfilling lives as they age.

Moreover, Dr. Cook's responsibilities go beyond dietary advice. She has constantly pushed for a holistic approach to wellbeing, highlighting the fact that physical activity, social connections, and emotional well-being are just as important to overall health as diet. Seniors like John, who have adopted an active lifestyle, enhanced their food choices, and developed deep social interactions, are clear examples of her effect.

Acknowledgment

This book is a tribute to the steadfast inspiration and support of many individuals who helped make this book possible. It has been a collaborative and labor-of-love endeavor.

We extend our sincere gratitude to the seniors who have shared their experiences, difficulties, and triumphs in their quest for improved health. Your fortitude and readiness to adopt a Mediterranean diet have served as an inspiration and a continual reminder of the transformational potential of constructive change.

We are grateful to the physicians, dietitians, and other nutrition specialists who have contributed their expertise, enabling us to guarantee that the data on these pages is based on the most recent findings and recommendations.

We would especially like to thank our friends and family for their unfailing support and encouragement during our adventure. This project has been developed on the foundation of your support.

We would like to express our gratitude to the users and readers of this book, whose commitment to their health and well-being is an example to all of us. This book has been written with you in mind, and your dedication to adopting a more energetic and healthy lifestyle is proof of the transformative potential of positive change.

In conclusion, we are delighted to deeply appreciate Dr. Angel Cook, the book's author, whose unwavering commitment, knowledge, and compassion have been the inspiration for our endeavor. Your work with elders has had a profoundly positive impact, and your dedication to making others' lives better is very remarkable.

This book is the result of many people working together, and we sincerely thank everyone who contributed. We hope that the rich flavors and wholesome traditions of the Mediterranean diet will continue to serve as a beacon for seniors seeking improved health and well-being.

With heartfelt gratitude,

The Group

INTRODUCTION

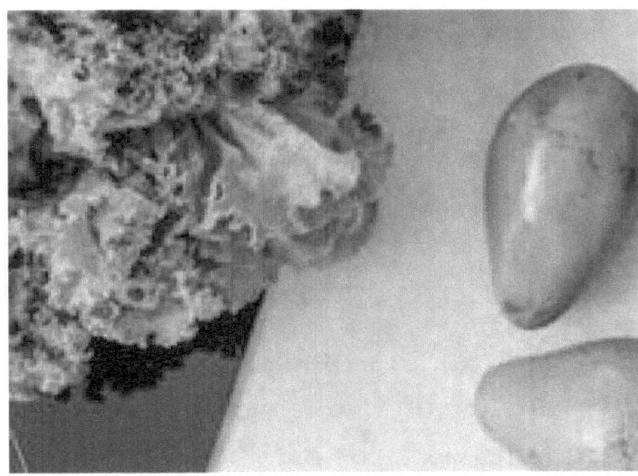

Welcome to a gastronomic voyage honoring the most meaningful moments in life. We encourage you to experience the mouthwatering rich flavors, vivid colors, and nutritious delights of the Mediterranean diet—a nurturing and ageless eating style that spans generations—in the pages of this cookbook.

It becomes even more crucial to carefully and wisely nourish our bodies as we gracefully enter our golden years.

For decades, the Mediterranean diet has been highly regarded for its ability to enhance vitality and overall health. It provides seniors with a sense of purpose and grace when navigating the nutritional landscape.

We set out on a journey that sounds as tasty as it does on these pages. The Mediterranean diet is a philosophy that honors the diversity of life rather than just a manner of eating. It combines the wisdom of centuries of culinary heritage with the pleasure of sharing meals and the art of appreciating healthful, sun-kissed ingredients.

This diet helps seniors maintain their health, manage chronic diseases, and live a life full of flavor, connection, and enjoyment by emphasizing fresh fruits and vegetables, whole grains, lean proteins, and heart-healthy fats.

Starting with the fundamentals, we will explore the vibrant tapestry of Mediterranean food, which spans from the sun-drenched fields of Spain to the serene coastlines of Italy and Greece. We will explore the diverse range of products, spices, and herbs that combine to create a feast for the senses in Mediterranean cookery.

You'll find a plentiful crop of dishes that have been carefully chosen with elders in mind throughout this cookbook. There's no shortage of inspiration here, whether you're new to the Mediterranean diet or have been following it for a while — from easy yet delicious breakfasts to leisurely and filling meals. Every dish is designed to nurture your spirit as much as your body.

In the kitchen, we are aware of the special requirements and preferences of the elderly. For this reason, we've filled these pages with useful tips on portion control, essential kitchen tools and utensils, tips for dining out, and tips for grocery shopping and meal planning.

But the joy of eating with family and friends is what the Mediterranean diet is all about, not simply what's on your plate. We appreciate the social element of dining together, which can create long-lasting connections and strengthen ties.

Since a Mediterranean diet has traditionally been linked to health and longevity, we hope this cookbook will provide you with the tools you need to start writing the next delectable chapter of your life. We cordially welcome you to peruse these pages with an open mind and an inquisitive palate, setting out on a gastronomic journey that guarantees not just better days but also happier ones.

So get ready to go off on a culinary adventure full of delectable meals, shared giggles, and treasured moments, regardless of your level of experience in the kitchen. It's a journey of exploration as well as a celebration of health, love, and life.

Welcome to the Mediterranean Diet Cookbook for Seniors 2024, a timeless blend of flavor, customs, and elegance to adorn your table and uplift your soul.

A Brief Overview Of The Mediterranean Diet

The Mediterranean diet, renowned for its health benefits and culinary delights, transcends mere dietary choices; it embodies a way of life. Anchored in the wholesome traditions of the Mediterranean region, it champions the consumption of fresh, vibrant produce, whole grains, and healthy fats.

The diet is characterized by the bountiful use of fruits, vegetables, and olive oil, complemented by whole grains like quinoa and brown rice. Lean proteins, with a focus on fatty fish and moderation in red meat consumption, are key components. Legumes, nuts, and a rich tapestry of herbs and spices infuse every dish with flavor and nutrition. Meals are savored with friends and family, reflecting a social dining tradition that emphasizes the joy of shared moments.

Beyond the plate, the Mediterranean lifestyle encourages moderation in wine consumption, an appreciation of local and seasonal ingredients, and the art of eating slowly and mindfully. This dietary pattern has been associated with numerous health benefits, including improved heart health, weight management, and a reduced risk of chronic diseases, offering not just sustenance but a pathway to a longer and more vibrant life. What sets it apart is its adaptability, making it accessible and enjoyable for a diverse range of individuals.

THE MEDITERRANEAN DIET'S BENEFITS

Recent research, featured in the journal JAMA Internal Medicine, highlights the significant benefits of seniors embracing the Mediterranean diet. This dietary approach has been linked to a decreased risk of mortality from various causes, encompassing heart disease, stroke, and cancer. Notably, the findings also underscore a reduced likelihood of developing dementia and Alzheimer's disease among seniors who adhere to the Mediterranean diet.

Moreover, another study published in the journal Neurology has shed light on the positive impact of this diet on brain health. Seniors who maintain a Mediterranean diet tend to exhibit a better-preserved hippocampus, a critical brain region responsible for memory and learning. This dietary pattern is not only associated with a diminished risk of cognitive decline but also offers protection against the onset of dementia.

In essence, these studies underscore the Mediterranean diet as an exceptional choice for seniors, offering a wealth of health benefits. It serves as a nutritional foundation that reduces the risk of chronic illnesses and contributes to an enhanced state of overall well-being.

With so many advantages for older adults, the Mediterranean diet is a widely recommended nutritional pattern. Among the principal advantages are the following ones:

Heart Health:

The heart-protective properties of the Mediterranean diet are well known. Reduced risks of heart disease, high blood pressure, and high cholesterol — all typical concerns as people age — benefit seniors. Cardiovascular health is supported by the diet's concentration on heart-healthy fats like almonds and olive oil as well as the eating of fatty seafood like salmon.

Cognitive Health:

Research indicates that a Mediterranean diet may help protect against cognitive decline and neurodegenerative illnesses like Alzheimer's while also maintaining cognitive function. One important factor supporting brain health is the high concentration of antioxidants found in fruits, vegetables, and whole grains.

Weight Management:

Because of changes in metabolism, seniors may find it more difficult to maintain a healthy weight. The Mediterranean diet promotes nutrient-dense eating, portion control, and satiety from foods high in fiber, all of which can help with weight management.

Bone Health:

The diet's emphasis on leafy greens, nuts, and dairy products — foods high in calcium — supports bone health by lowering the incidence of fractures and osteoporosis, two conditions that are frequent in later life.

Gut Health:

The high-fiber foods found in the Mediterranean diet, such as fruits, vegetables, and whole grains, help to maintain gut health. Better general health and a lower incidence of gastrointestinal problems are associated with a balanced gut flora.

Inflammation Reduction:

Numerous age-related illnesses are linked to chronic inflammation. Anti-inflammatory elements of the Mediterranean diet, such as antioxidants from fruits and vegetables and omega-3 fatty acids from fish, aid in the fight against inflammation.

Better Digestion:

Including foods high in fiber and fermented dairy products, such as Greek yogurt, in the diet helps to support digestive health, which lessens constipation and fosters a healthy gut.

Stable Blood Sugar:

The Mediterranean diet's focus on whole grains, legumes, and low-glycemic-index foods can help seniors with diabetes or those at risk maintain stable blood sugar levels and lessen their need for medication.

Eye Health:

A diet high in antioxidants, especially from foods like kale, spinach, and vibrant fruits, helps maintain eye health and may lower the risk of macular degeneration brought on by aging.

Lower Chance of Depression:

Seniors may be more susceptible to mood disorders and depression. The omega-3 fatty acids and nutrient-dense foods found in the Mediterranean diet have been linked to a decreased risk of depression and an improvement in mental health.

Social and Emotional Well-Being:

Eating together and maintaining a diet high in scrumptious, fresh foods can improve general happiness, create a sense of community, and strengthen social ties, all of which can lessen feelings of isolation and loneliness.

Longevity:

Studies on the Mediterranean diet have shown that people live longer and are more likely to be happy in their older years.

Decreased risk of chronic concerns:

Seniors who may already be managing certain health concerns may find special benefits from the diet's link to decreased chances of chronic diseases like diabetes, heart disease, and cancer.

Vitality and Energy:

The Mediterranean diet's emphasis on complete, nutrient-rich foods gives you the energy you need to be active as you age.

HOW TO USE THIS BOOK

This book is your pass on a voyage through the age-old customs of Mediterranean cuisine that offers health, flavor, and vibrancy. We want to make sure you get the most out of this book and incorporate the Mediterranean diet easily into your daily life as you set out on this gastronomic journey. To make the most of this book, follow these tips:

1. Start with the Introduction: To have a thorough understanding of the Mediterranean diet, its advantages for senior citizens, and what to anticipate from this book, start with reading the introduction. This section lays out the background information and your journey's objectives.

2. Get started with the basics: We've added sections with information like important food groups and the nutrients they require, portion sizes and their recommended daily intake for seniors who follow a Mediterranean diet and the advantages of doing so. These are excellent tools to improve your comprehension of and performance with the Mediterranean diet.

3. Look Around the Food Chart: A long list of foods that are recommended for the Mediterranean diet may be found in this area, including fruits, vegetables, whole grains, legumes, proteins, and more. This is the resource you should use the most while preparing wholesome, well-balanced meals.

4. Explore the dishes: This book's assortment of delectable Mediterranean dishes is its core. Look through the sections for breakfast, lunch, supper, and snacks to discover a range of options that fit your dietary requirements and preferences. Ingredient lists, comprehensive preparation directions, and nutritional data are included with every recipe.

5. 28-Day Meal Plan: We've created a 28-day meal plan that eliminates uncertainty about what to eat for people who appreciate structure. For four weeks, the meal plan provides a well-rounded and diverse assortment of Mediterranean-inspired dishes.

7. Make It Personal: You can customize the Mediterranean diet to fit your nutritional needs and tastes. Feel free to modify the recipes to your preferences, and if you have any questions about a particular diet, speak with your healthcare professional.

8. Keep Up to Date: Nutrition is a field that is constantly changing. Keep abreast of the most recent recommendations and health facts. We hope you will regularly refer back to this book to make sure your dietary decisions are in line with the most recent guidelines.

9. Share the Journey: You might want to take your loved ones along for this gastronomic journey. The social features of the Mediterranean diet can be strengthened by cooking and dining together, which promotes a sense of community and shared well-being.

10. Appreciate Your Progress: As you adopt a Mediterranean diet, stop to acknowledge and appreciate your accomplishments, no matter how small they may seem. It is important to celebrate each step you take to live a better, happier life.

You'll find lots of information, ideas, and delicious recipes on the pages that follow to help you along the path of the Mediterranean diet. It is our intention that this book becomes your reliable guide on the road to a healthier, more active senior life, regardless of how long you have been an enthusiast or how recently you have begun to investigate this lifestyle.

Now turn the pages, take a gastronomic tour, and enjoy the tastes, customs, and well-being that come with following a Mediterranean diet. I hope your journey to a happier, healthier senior life goes well. Good appetite!

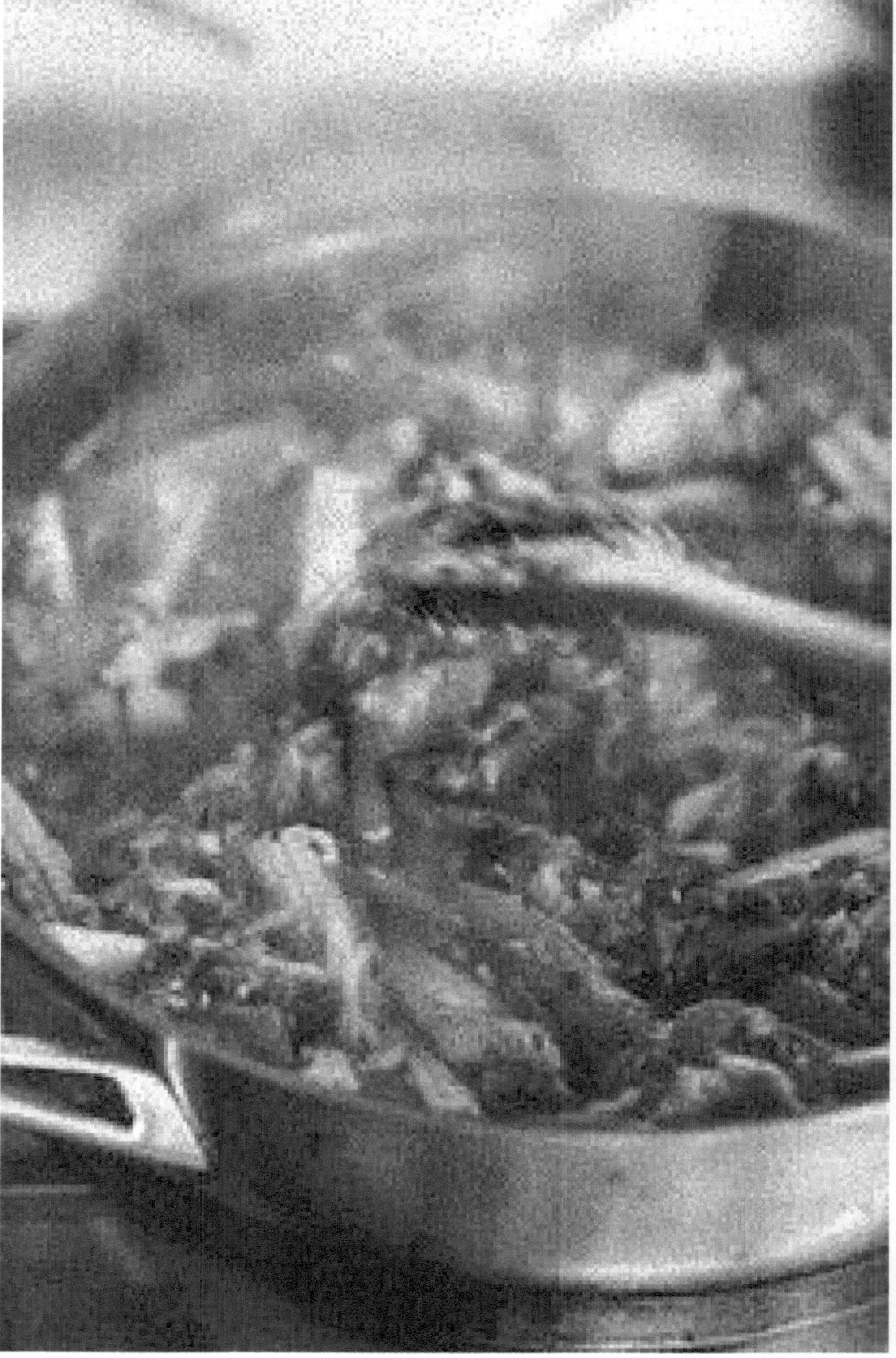

CHAPTER 1: THE BASICS

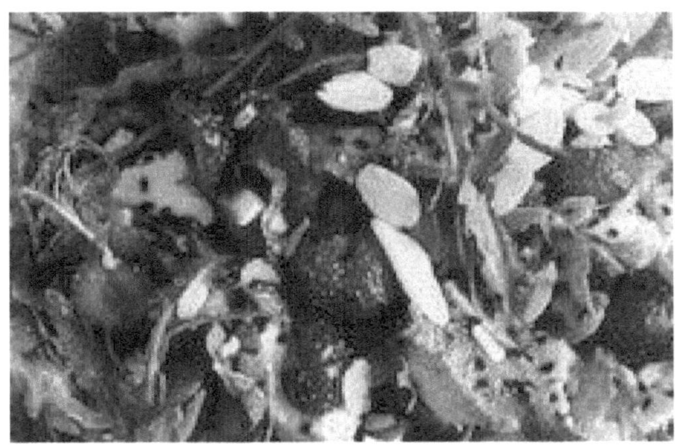

ESSENTIAL KITCHEN TOOLS AND UTENSILS

Anybody can benefit from having a well-stocked kitchen, but those on a Mediterranean diet really should. The following is a list of necessary kitchen appliances and utensils to assist you in preparing delectable Mediterranean meals:

- **Chef's Knife:** The most crucial instrument for dicing, slicing, and cutting a range of ingredients is a good chef's knife.

- **Paring Knife:** This little knife is ideal for finer work such as slicing, peeling, and trimming tiny fruits and vegetables.
- **Bread Knife:** Perfect for slicing through delicate pastries or crusty bread.
- **Serrated Knife:** Slice soft-skinned fruits like tomatoes and other vegetables with this knife without crushing them.
- **Cutting Board:** To keep your knives and counters safe, get a sturdy cutting board. Cutting boards made of plastic or wood are useful.
- **Vegetable Peeler:** An efficient instrument for fruit and vegetable peeling and trimming.
- **Grater:** For grating cheese, zest from citrus, and veggies like carrots and zucchini.
- **Mandoline Slicer:** Fruits and vegetables can be quickly and precisely sliced using a mandoline.
- **Kitchen shears:** These are useful for opening food packaging, trimming meats, and chopping herbs.
- **Measuring Spoons and Cups:** Make sure recipe measurements are correct.
- **Mixing Bowls:** You'll need bowls of different sizes for marinating, mixing ingredients, and keeping leftovers.
- **Whisk:** Excellent for mixing and whisking sauce and dressing ingredients.
- **Wooden Spatula:** To prevent scratching non-stick cookware, use this for stirring and sautéing.

- **Tongs:** Needed for rotating, flipping, and serving meals.
- **Slotted Spoon:** Helpful for serving and draining liquid-cooked meals.
- **A silicone spatula:** This is ideal for scraping the sides of pots and bowls to ensure that all of your delectable creations get consumed.
- **Colander:** An essential tool for straining legumes, washing veggies, and draining pasta.
- **Pepper Mill and Salt Shaker:** Mediterranean foods taste better when they are prepared with freshly ground pepper and sea salt.
- **Garlic Press**: Make chopping garlic easier for a variety of Mediterranean dishes.
- **Can opener:** used to open goods like beans and tomatoes that are canned.
- **21. Corkscrew:** If you want to pair your Mediterranean dinners with a glass of red wine.
- **22. Microplane/Zester:** For extra taste, grate cheese, spices, or citrus zest.
- **23. Salad Spinner:** Make sure your greens are well-cleaned and dehydrated before using them in salads.
- **24. Baking sheets and pans:** These are necessary for making Mediterranean pastries and roasting veggies.
- **25. Saucepan and Pot:** Use various sizes while preparing pasta, grains, and sauces.
- **26. Dutch Oven:** Excellent for Mediterranean one-pot meals and stews that cook slowly.

- **27. Food processors or blenders:** These are great for creating sauces, dips, and smoothies.
- **28. Grill or Grill Pan:** Ideal for Mediterranean-style grilled foods such as veggies and kebabs.
- **29. Oven mitts:** to shield your hands from hot cookware.
- **30. Food Storage Containers:** Make sure you have a range of containers for meal planning and keeping leftovers.

IMPORTANT FOOD GROUPS AND THE NUTRITIONAL ADVANTAGES

The main food groups in the Mediterranean diet each have unique nutritional advantages:

Vegetables and fruits:

This group is rich in antioxidants, minerals, and vitamins. Vitamin C is found in fruits like berries and citrus, whereas vitamin K is found in leafy greens. Tomatoes and bell peppers are two colorful veggies that are high in vitamins A and C. Additionally, the dietary fiber in these foods promotes healthy digestion and general well-being.

Whole Grains:

Complex carbohydrates and fiber are found in foods like whole wheat, brown rice, and quinoa, which help with digestion and maintain stable energy levels. They also include minerals and important B vitamins.

Legumes:

High in protein and a great source of dietary fiber are beans, lentils, and chickpeas. They are necessary for general health because they supply iron, folate, and key amino acids.

Lean Proteins:

Omega-3 fatty acids, which are good for the heart, are found in fish, especially fatty types like salmon and mackerel. Turkey and other poultry provide lean protein. Eggs are an excellent source of important minerals including vitamin D and choline as well as protein.

Dairy and Dairy Alternatives:

Cheese and Greek yogurt provide calcium and protein. Almond and soy milk are supplemented with vital vitamins and minerals for individuals who prefer them to dairy products.

Nuts and Seeds:

Rich sources of protein, healthy fats, and a variety of vitamins and minerals are almonds, walnuts, and flaxseeds. They have a high concentration of polyunsaturated and monounsaturated fats.

Healthy Fats:

Extra virgin olive oil is the traditional Mediterranean fat, valued for its antioxidant and heart-healthy monounsaturated fats. It is a necessary part of the diet. Another good source of fats is avocado.

Herbs and Spices:

Herbs such as oregano, rosemary, and thyme contribute phytonutrients and antioxidants while imparting taste without the need for added salt. Not only can spices like paprika and cumin improve flavor, but they may also have health advantages.

Fish and seafood:

Fish provides high-quality protein and is good for the heart, especially when it contains omega-3 fatty acids.

Wine (in moderation):

Red wine contains substances like resveratrol, which may have some heart-protective effects when ingested in moderation.

PORTION SIZES AND THEIR RECOMMENDED DAILY INTAKE

Seniors' recommended daily consumption and portion sizes may change based on their specific nutritional demands, activity levels, and medical conditions. However, the following basic recommendations for seniors' daily consumption and portion sizes for the major food groups in the Mediterranean diet are:

Fruits and Vegetables:

- Portion Size: 1 cup of raw or 1/2 cup of cooked

vegetables; 1 medium-sized fruit.

- Daily Intake: Aim for 5-9 servings of fruits and vegetables daily, with a variety of colors and types to ensure a wide range of nutrients.

Whole Grains:

- **Portion Size:** 1/2 cup of cooked grains (rice, quinoa, bulgur); 1 slice of whole wheat bread.
- **Daily Intake:** Include 6-8 servings of whole grains in your daily meals for sustained energy and fiber.

Legumes:

- Portion Size: 1/2 cup of cooked beans or lentils.
- Daily Intake: Aim for at least 2-3 servings per week to provide essential protein and dietary fiber.

Lean Proteins:

- Portion Size: 3-4 ounces of cooked fish or poultry; 2 eggs; 1-2 ounces of cheese.
- Daily Intake: Include fish 2-3 times a week and poultry or eggs as preferred sources of protein.

Dairy and Dairy Alternatives:

- Portion Size: 1 cup of milk or yogurt; 1.5 ounces of cheese.
- Daily Intake: 2-3 servings of dairy or dairy alternatives to support calcium and protein intake.

Nuts and Seeds:

- Portion Size: 1 ounce of nuts or seeds (about a small handful).
- Daily Intake: Enjoy a small portion as a snack or add to salads, aiming for 2-3 servings per week.

Healthy Fats:

- Portion Size: 1-2 tablespoons of extra virgin olive oil.
- Daily Intake: Use olive oil as your primary cooking fat and source of healthy fats.

Herbs and Spices:

- Portion Size: Use freely to enhance flavor without specific portion guidelines.

Fish and Seafood:

- Portion Size: 3-4 ounces of cooked fish or seafood.
- Daily Intake: Include fish 2-3 times a week, especially fatty fish like salmon.

Wine (in moderation):

- Portion Size: Up to 5 ounces (a small glass) for women and up to 10 ounces for men daily.
- Daily Intake: Limit wine to moderate consumption based on individual preferences and health considerations.

CHAPTER 2: GETTING STARTED

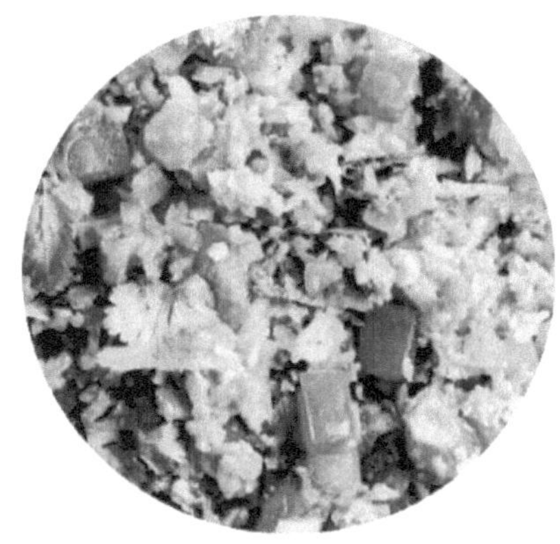

HOW TO FOLLOW THE MEDITERRANEAN DIET AS A SENIOR

If you're a senior looking to adopt the Mediterranean diet, explained below are some practical guidelines to help you get started:

1. Prioritize Plant-Based Foods: Make sure a substantial portion of your meals consists of fruits, vegetables, whole grains, and legumes.
2. Opt for Healthy Fats: Select olive oil or avocado oil as your primary sources of dietary fat.

3. Reduce Red Meat and Processed Meats: Limit your intake of red meat to no more than once a week and avoid processed meats entirely.
4. Include Fish Twice a Week: Fish is an excellent source of omega-3 fatty acids, which promote heart health and cognitive function. Aim to incorporate it into your diet at least twice a week.
5. Consume Dairy Products in Moderation: Opt for low-fat or fat-free dairy options like yogurt and cheese, enjoying them in sensible portions.
6. Minimize Sugary Beverages and Sweets: Make water your primary beverage choice, reducing your consumption of sugary drinks and sweets for better overall health.

How to Adapt the Mediterranean Diet to Different Individual Needs

For Seniors with Limited Mobility or Dexterity:

- Opt for pre-cut fruits and vegetables for convenience.
- Consider frozen meals or quick-heating meal options.
- Utilize kitchen appliances like food processors or slow cookers to simplify meal preparation.

For Seniors with Diabetes:

- Focus on low-glycemic foods such as whole grains, legumes, and vegetables.

- Restrict consumption of sugary beverages and sweets.
- Maintain stable blood sugar levels by consuming regular meals and snacks throughout the day.

For Seniors with High Blood Pressure:

- Choose low-sodium foods like fresh fruits, vegetables, whole grains, and lean protein sources.
- Minimize intake of processed foods, canned items, and high-sodium dishes.

For Seniors with High Cholesterol:

- Opt for foods low in saturated and trans fats, including lean protein sources, fruits, vegetables, and whole grains.
- Limit red meat, processed meats, and full-fat dairy products in your diet.

For Seniors with Kidney Issues:

- If you have kidney problems, your healthcare provider may recommend restricting protein intake. Opt for lower-protein sources such as fish, poultry, and plant-based proteins like legumes, and limit high-protein foods like red meat.
- Kidney issues can affect the body's ability to regulate phosphorus and potassium levels. Reduce phosphorus intake by avoiding processed foods, colas, and foods high in phosphate additives. Similarly, manage potassium by limiting high-

potassium foods like bananas, oranges, and tomatoes.

- Reducing salt and sodium intake can help manage blood pressure and fluid balance. Choose fresh foods and season with herbs and spices instead of salt.

TIPS FOR GROCERY SHOPPING AND MEAL PLANNING

Organizing meals and doing your grocery shopping are crucial to implementing the Mediterranean diet. The following advice will help you get the most out of your grocery shopping and meal planning:

Planning Meals:

- **Make sensible goals:** Establish your nutritional objectives, such as increasing the number of fruits and vegetables in your diet, cutting back on saturated fats, or closely adhering to the Mediterranean diet.
- **Make a Meal Plan:** Make a menu for the next week. A range of Mediterranean-inspired breakfast, lunch, supper, and snack options should be included. This promotes variety and a balanced diet.
- **Use Seasonal Vegetables:** Select in-season fruits and vegetables. They are typically less priced, more tasty, and fresher.

- **Balanced Macronutrients:** Make sure your meals include a healthy proportion of fats, proteins, and carbohydrates. The balance of the Mediterranean diet is well-known.

- **Batch Cooking:** Make bigger batches of food and store individual servings in the freezer for later. This facilitates diet adherence, particularly on hectic days.

- **Ingenious Use of Leftovers:** Incorporate leftovers into fresh recipes. Roasted veggies, for instance, work well in salads or as the base for a frittata.

- **Mindful Eating:** Engage in mindful eating by appreciating the social aspects of meals, savoring every bite, and being aware of your body's signals of hunger and fullness.

Food Shopping:

- **Make a list of things to buy**: Make a thorough shopping list based on your food plan. This guarantees you have everything you need and helps you avoid making impulsive purchases.

- **Shop the Periphery:** Fresh produce, dairy products, and meats are typically found on the periphery of grocery shops. If you're looking for Mediterranean components, concentrate on these parts.

- **Read Labels:** Look for added sugars, trans fats, and sodium on product labels. Select goods that have undergone little processing or additions.

- **Purchase Whole Grains:** Choose whole-grain products such as brown rice and whole wheat pasta. Find the term "whole" in the list of ingredients.
- **Pick Lean Proteins:** Go for skinless chicken and lean meat cuts. Include plant-based proteins like legumes and tofu.
- **Accept Fresh Herbs:** To enhance the flavor of your food, purchase fresh herbs like thyme, basil, and oregano. They are essential to Mediterranean cuisine.
- **Stock Up on Extra Virgin Olive Oil:** Make a purchase of this oil. It's an essential ingredient in Mediterranean cuisine and a good source of fats.
- **Frozen Fruits and Vegetables:** These are convenient and frequently equally as nutrient-dense as their fresh counterparts. They perform admirably in numerous recipes.
- **Buy in Bulk:** To save money, buy non-perishable basics like beans, whole grains, and canned tomatoes in large quantities.
- **Try Something New:** To add some variety to your diet, try some new Mediterranean foods like tahini, fennel, or artichokes.
- **Steer clear of Impulse Purchases:** Follow your shopping list and refrain from making impulsive purchases.
- **Minimize Food Waste:** Arrange meals so that ingredients are used up before going bad. Make inventive use of leftovers and think about composting.

TIPS FOR DINING OUT

Eating out may be both nourishing and pleasurable when adhering to a Mediterranean diet. To help you enjoy your meal to the fullest, consider these suggestions:

- **Select Mediterranean Dining Establishments:** Choose Mediterranean or similar specialty restaurants since their menus are more likely to have diet-friendly options.
- **Examine the Menu Ahead of Time:** A lot of eateries now offer their menus online. To ensure you make well-informed decisions, take some time to browse over the menu.
- **Begin with a Salad:** Get your meal started with a crisp salad. Request a dressing of olive oil, vinegar, or lemon juice. Steer clear of cream dressings.
- **Choose Baked or Grilled:** Rather than frying, opt for baked, roasted, or grilled foods. As a result, there are fewer additional fats.
- **Put an Emphasis on Seafood:** Fish and seafood are staples of Mediterranean cooking. Try ordering grilled shrimp, mackerel, or salmon.
- **Pick Whole Grains:** If at all feasible, request meals that include whole grains, such as bulgur, quinoa, or whole wheat pasta.
- **Fill Up on Veggies:** Mediterranean cuisine is known for its abundance of veggies. Choose recipes that have an abundance of vibrant vegetables, and think about getting a side order of grilled veggies.

- **Regulate servings:** Food servings in restaurants can be generous. If you have leftovers, think about splitting a dish with a dining companion or asking for a to-go container.
- **Limit Red Meat:** Although the Mediterranean diet calls for moderate consumption of red meat, when you do order beef or lamb meals, try to select thin cuts.
- **Request Sauces on the Side:** Mediterranean dips and sauces may have a lot of calories. Use them sparingly and ask for them on the side.
- **Select Legumes:** Chickpeas and lentils are frequently used in Mediterranean cuisine. Consider choices like chickpea hummus or lentil soup.
- **Savor Olives:** An essential component of Mediterranean cooking, olives can enhance the flavor and nutritional value of your food.
- **Pay Attention to Bread:** If bread is provided before dinner, eat it sparingly. Go ahead and choose whole-grain bread.
- **Don't Overindulge in Sweets:** Mediterranean sweets can be decadent. If there is a fruit-based dessert choice, select it or share it with the people at the table.
- **Stay Hydrated:** Choose unsweetened herbal tea or water to go with your meal. Wine should be consumed in moderation if you drink alcohol.
- **Request Modifications:** Do not be afraid to request changes to accommodate your dietary requirements. The majority of eateries are welcoming.

CHAPTER 3: FITNESS AND DIETING

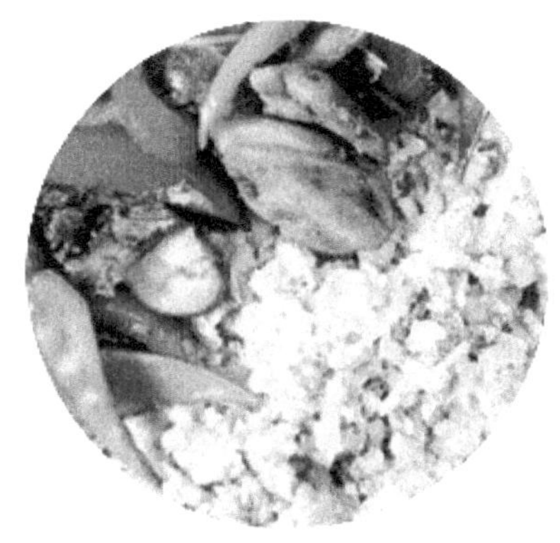

FOOD LISTS

Fruits:

- Apples
- Oranges
- Bananas
- Berries (strawberries, blueberries, raspberries)
- Grapes
- Pomegranates
- Citrus fruits (lemons, limes)

- Melons (watermelon, cantaloupe)
- Cherries
- Figs
- Kiwifruit
- Avocado
- Peaches
- Apricots
- Plums
- Nectarines
- Mangoes
- Pineapples
- Papayas
- Dates

Vegetables:

- Tomatoes
- Cucumbers
- Bell peppers
- Onions
- Garlic
- Spinach
- Kale
- Swiss chard
- Broccoli
- Cauliflower
- Zucchini
- Eggplant
- Artichokes
- Asparagus

- Brussels sprouts
- Celery
- Green leafy lettuce
- Radicchio
- Radishes
- Cabbage
- Carrots
- Beets
- Green beans
- Peas
- Squash (acorn, butternut, etc.)
- Leeks
- Scallions
- Turnips
- Mushrooms
- Okra
- Cress
- Arugula
- Watercress
- Endive
- Parsnips
- Sweet potatoes
- Swiss chard
- Mustard greens
- Collard greens

Whole Grains:

- Whole wheat bread
- Whole wheat pasta

- Brown rice
- Bulgur
- Quinoa
- Farro
- Oats
- Barley
- Whole grain couscous
- Millet
- Teff

Legumes:

- Chickpeas
- Lentils
- Black beans
- White beans
- Fava beans
- Peas
- Mung beans
- Cannellini beans
- Kidney beans
- Lima beans
- Garbanzo beans

Nuts and Seeds:

- Almonds
- Walnuts
- Pistachios
- Cashews
- Sunflower seeds

- Chia seeds
- Flaxseeds
- Pumpkin seeds
- Sesame seeds

Proteins:

- Fish (salmon, tuna, sardines, mackerel, trout)
- Poultry (chicken, turkey)
- Eggs
- Greek yogurt
- Low-fat or non-fat milk
- Plant-based milk alternatives (almond, soy, oat, coconut)
- Tofu
- Tempeh
- Seitan
- Hummus

Dairy and Dairy Alternatives:

- Feta cheese
- Goat cheese
- Greek yogurt
- Low-fat or non-fat yogurt
- Ricotta cheese
- Parmesan cheese
- Plant-based cheese alternatives

Oils and Fats:

- Extra virgin olive oil

- Nuts and seeds oils (walnut oil, flaxseed oil)
- Avocado oil
- Canola oil

Herbs and Spices:

- Basil
- Oregano
- Rosemary
- Thyme
- Mint
- Cilantro
- Dill
- Parsley
- Cinnamon
- Cumin
- Coriander
- Paprika
- Turmeric
- Saffron
- Bay leaves

Beverages:

- Water
- Herbal teas
- Green tea
- Red wine (in moderation)
- Coffee

Sweets (in moderation):

- Honey
- Dark chocolate (70% cocoa or higher)

Condiments:

- Balsamic vinegar
- Red wine vinegar
- Lemon juice
- Tahini
- Tzatziki
- Pesto

Seafood:

- Shrimp
- Calamari
- Clams
- Mussels
- Crab
- Lobster
- Scallops

Poultry:

- Duck
- Quail
- Turkey breast

Red Meat (in moderation):

- Lean cuts of beef (sirloin, tenderloin)
- Lamb

Dried Herbs:

- Herbes de Provence
- Za'atar
- Garam masala
- Curry powder
- Chili powder
- Paprika

MEAL PLAN

Day 1:

- **Breakfast**: Mediterranean Omelette
- **Lunch**: Greek Salad with Grilled Chicken
- **Dinner**: Grilled Lemon Herb Chicken
- **Snack**: Hummus with Veggies

Day 2:

- **Breakfast**: Greek Yogurt Parfait
- **Lunch**: Mediterranean Tuna Salad
- **Dinner**: Ratatouille
- **Snack**: Greek Yogurt topped with Nuts and Honey

Day 3:

- **Breakfast**: Shakshuka
- **Lunch**: Panzanella Salad
- **Dinner**: Mediterranean Baked Salmon
- **Snack**: Mediterranean Olives and Cheese Platter

Day 4:

- **Breakfast**: Ful Medames
- **Lunch**: Mediterranean Stuffed Peppers
- **Dinner**: Paella
- **Snack**: Mediterranean Cucumber Cups

Day 5:

- **Breakfast**: Mediterranean Breakfast Salad
- **Lunch**: Mediterranean Baked Sea Bass
- **Dinner**: Lamb Moussaka
- **Snack**: Mediterranean Sardine Toast

Day 6:

- **Breakfast**: Labneh and Za'atar Toast
- **Lunch**: Mediterranean Vegetable Stew
- **Dinner**: Shrimp Scampi
- **Snack**: Mediterranean Feta and Watermelon Bites

Day 7:

- **Breakfast**: Spanakopita
- **Lunch**: Grilled Lemon Herb Chicken
- **Dinner**: Mediterranean Baked Salmon
- **Snack**: Stuffed Dates with Almonds

Week 2:

Day 8:

- **Breakfast**: Mediterranean Chia Pudding
- **Lunch**: Greek Salad with Grilled Chicken

- **Dinner**: Ratatouille
- **Snack**: Hummus with Veggies

Day 9:

- **Breakfast**: Greek Yogurt Parfait
- **Lunch**: Mediterranean Tuna Salad
- **Dinner**: Paella
- **Snack**: Greek Yogurt topped with Nuts and Honey

Day 10:

- **Breakfast**: Shakshuka
- **Lunch**: Panzanella Salad
- **Dinner**: Mediterranean Baked Sea Bass
- **Snack**: Mediterranean Olives and Cheese Platter

Day 11:

- **Breakfast**: Ful Medames
- **Lunch**: Mediterranean Stuffed Peppers
- **Dinner**: Shrimp Scampi
- **Snack**: Mediterranean Cucumber Cups

Day 12:

- **Breakfast**: Mediterranean Breakfast Salad
- **Lunch**: Mediterranean Vegetable Stew
- **Dinner**: Mediterranean Stuffed Peppers
- **Snack**: Mediterranean Sardine Toast

Day 13:

- **Breakfast**: Labneh and Za'atar Toast
- **Lunch**: Mediterranean Tuna Salad

- **Dinner**: Grilled Lemon Herb Chicken
- **Snack**: Mediterranean Feta and Watermelon Bites

Day 14:

- **Breakfast**: Spanakopita
- **Lunch**: Greek Salad with Grilled Chicken
- **Dinner**: Lamb Moussaka
- **Snack**: Stuffed Dates with Almonds

Week 3:

Day 15:

- **Breakfast**: Mediterranean Chia Pudding
- **Lunch**: Panzanella Salad
- **Dinner**: Mediterranean Baked Salmon
- **Snack**: Hummus with Veggies

Day 16:

- **Breakfast**: Greek Yogurt Parfait
- **Lunch**: Mediterranean Tuna Salad
- **Dinner**: Ratatouille
- **Snack**: Greek Yogurt topped with Nuts and Honey

Day 17:

- **Breakfast**: Shakshuka
- **Lunch**: Mediterranean Baked Sea Bass
- **Dinner**: Paella
- **Snack**: Mediterranean Olives and Cheese Platter

Day 18:

- **Breakfast**: Ful Medames
- **Lunch**: Mediterranean Stuffed Peppers
- **Dinner**: Shrimp Scampi
- **Snack**: Mediterranean Cucumber Cups

Day 19:

- **Breakfast**: Mediterranean Breakfast Salad
- **Lunch**: Mediterranean Vegetable Stew
- **Dinner**: Mediterranean Stuffed Peppers
- **Snack**: Mediterranean Sardine Toast

Day 20:

- **Breakfast**: Labneh and Za'atar Toast
- **Lunch**: Mediterranean Tuna Salad
- **Dinner**: Grilled Lemon Herb Chicken
- **Snack**: Mediterranean Feta and Watermelon Bites

Day 21:

- **Breakfast**: Spanakopita
- **Lunch**: Greek Salad with Grilled Chicken
- **Dinner**: Lamb Moussaka
- **Snack**: Stuffed Dates with Almonds

Week 4:

Day 22:

- **Breakfast**: Mediterranean Chia Pudding
- **Lunch**: Panzanella Salad
- **Dinner**: Mediterranean Baked Salmon
- **Snack**: Hummus with Veggies

Day 23:

- **Breakfast**: Greek Yogurt Parfait
- **Lunch**: Mediterranean Tuna Salad
- **Dinner**: Paella
- **Snack**: Greek Yogurt topped with Nuts and Honey

Day 24:

- **Breakfast**: Shakshuka
- **Lunch**: Mediterranean Baked Sea Bass
- **Dinner**: Mediterranean Vegetable Stew
- **Snack**: Mediterranean Olives and Cheese Platter

Day 25:

- **Breakfast**: Ful Medames
- **Lunch**: Mediterranean Stuffed Peppers
- **Dinner**: Shrimp Scampi
- **Snack**: Mediterranean Cucumber Cups

Day 26:

- **Breakfast**: Mediterranean Breakfast Salad
- **Lunch**: Mediterranean Vegetable Stew
- **Dinner**: Mediterranean Stuffed Peppers
- **Snack**: Mediterranean Sardine Toast

Day 27:

- **Breakfast**: Labneh and Za'atar Toast
- **Lunch**: Mediterranean Tuna Salad
- **Dinner**: Grilled Lemon Herb Chicken
- **Snack**: Mediterranean Feta and Watermelon Bites

Day 28:

- **Breakfast**: Spanakopita
- **Lunch**: Greek Salad with Grilled Chicken
- **Dinner**: Lamb Moussaka
- **Snack**: Stuffed Dates with Almonds

PHYSICAL ACTIVITIES FOR SENIORS

For seniors, physical activity is a vital part of a healthy lifestyle. Frequent exercise maintains balance, improves mobility, elevates mood, and improves general well-being. Senior-friendly physical activities include the following:

- **Walking**: For seniors, walking is one of the finest low-impact workouts. It is simple, portable, and doesn't require any specialized tools. Most days of the week, try to get in at least 30 minutes of brisk walking.
- **Yoga:** Yoga is a great way to increase strength, flexibility, and balance. It also encourages mental health and relaxation. Seek out senior-focused classes or do mild yoga at home.
- **Tai Chi:** This slow-moving, flowing martial technique places a strong emphasis on synchronization and balance. Seniors can benefit most from it because it lowers their chance of falling.
- **Swimming:** Both swimming and water aerobics offer a full-body workout that is easy on the joints.

Water is a great option for people with arthritis or joint discomfort since it supports the body.

- **Strength Training:** To increase bone density and muscular tone, incorporate strength training activities with modest weights or resistance bands. Pay attention to exercises that work for the main muscle groups.
- **Cycling:** Using a standard cycle with the appropriate modifications or a stationary bike is a great approach to increasing leg strength and cardiovascular fitness. It is low-impact and adaptable to any person's degree of fitness.
- **Dancing:** Keeping active with dance is enjoyable. Dancing, be it ballroom, line, or just around the house, enhances balance and coordination.
- **Chair Exercises:** Chair exercises are a practical choice for people with restricted mobility. Maintaining muscle strength can be aided with seated marches, arm circles, and leg lifts.
- **Pilates:** Pilates emphasizes posture, flexibility, and core strength. Seniors can exercise gently and effectively with it.
- **Gardening:** Keeping active outside can be achieved through gardening. You may work out your entire body by digging, planting, pulling weeds, and caring for plants.
- **Golf:** Seniors can enjoy the outdoors and get some mild exercise by playing golf, which is a low-impact sport. Just be aware of how much walking is required.

- **Stair Climbing:** If you have access to a staircase, this easy exercise will help increase cardiovascular fitness and lower body strength. Use a railing for safety and proceed with caution.
- **Stretching:** Regular stretches help reduce stiffness in the muscles and increase flexibility. To preserve your range of motion, gently stretch your key muscle groups.
- **Balance exercises:** These can assist in maintaining stability and preventing falls. Examples of balance exercises include standing on one foot and utilizing a balancing board.
- **Group sessions:** You might want to enroll in senior-specific group exercise sessions. Numerous exercises, such as aerobics, strength training, and flexibility training, are frequently included in these programs.

CHAPTER 4: EASY DELECTABLE RECIPES

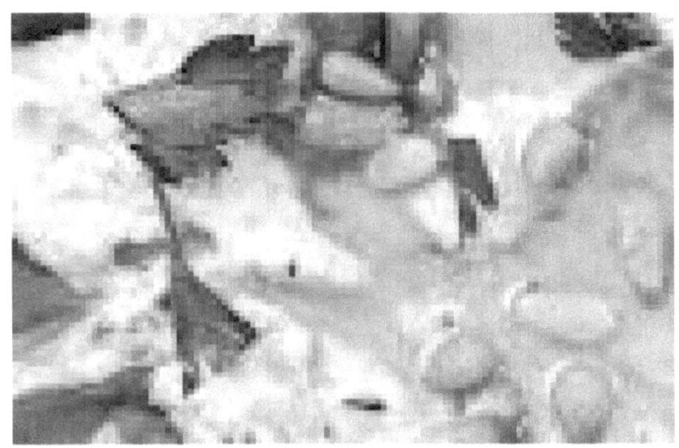

BREAKFAST:

Mediterranean Omelette:

Prep Time: 10 minutes

Ingredients:

- 2 eggs
- 2 tablespoons crumbled feta cheese
- 2 tablespoons diced tomatoes

- 1 tablespoon fresh herbs (e.g., basil, oregano)
- Olives and pita bread for serving

Instructions:

1. Whisk the eggs in a bowl until well-beaten.
2. Heat a non-stick pan over medium heat and add a little olive oil.
3. Pour the eggs into the pan and let them set for a minute.
4. Sprinkle feta, tomatoes, and herbs over one half of the omelette.
5. Fold the other half over the filling, creating a half-moon shape.
6. Cook for another 2-3 minutes until the omelette is cooked through.
7. Serve with olives and pita bread on the side.

Nutrient Information: Approximate values per serving (excluding olives and pita): Calories: 220, Protein: 14g, Fat: 16g, Carbohydrates: 5g, Fiber: 1g.

Greek Yogurt Parfait:

Prep Time: 5 minutes

Ingredients:

- 1 cup Greek yogurt
- 2 tablespoons honey
- 1/4 cup granola

- 1/2 cup of fresh berries, such as blueberries and strawberries

Instructions:

1. Arrange the Greek yogurt in a bowl or glass container.
2. Drizzle honey over the yogurt.
3. Sprinkle granola on top.
4. Add fresh berries.
5. Repeat the layering if desired.

Nutrient Information: Approximate values per serving: Calories: 320, Protein: 15g, Fat: 10g, Carbohydrates: 45g, Fiber: 5g.

Shakshuka

Prep Time: 15 minutes

Ingredients:

- 2 tablespoons olive oil
- 1 onion, diced
- 1 red bell pepper, diced
- 2 cloves garlic, minced
- 1 can (14 oz) crushed tomatoes
- 1 teaspoon ground cumin
- 1 teaspoon paprika
- Salt and pepper to taste
- 4 large eggs
- Fresh herbs (e.g., cilantro, parsley) for garnish

Instructions:

- Melt olive oil in a pan over moderate flame.
- Put the red pepper and onions, and saute until tender.
- Add salt, pepper, paprika, cumin, and garlic to the mixture.
- Pour in crushed tomatoes and simmer for 10 minutes.
- Create small wells in the tomato mixture and crack the eggs into them.
- Cook the eggs for about five minutes, covered, or until they set.
- Garnish with fresh herbs and serve.

Nutrient Information: Approximate values per serving (1/4 of the recipe): Calories: 230, Protein: 11g, Fat: 14g, Carbohydrates: 17g, Fiber: 4g.

Ful Medames

Prep Time: 15 minutes

Ingredients:

- 1 can (15 oz) fava beans
- 2 cloves garlic, minced
- 2 tablespoons olive oil
- Juice of 1 lemon
- Salt and cumin to taste
- Flatbread for serving

Instructions:

1. Drain and rinse the fava beans.
2. In a bowl, mash the fava beans with garlic, olive oil, lemon juice, salt, and cumin.
3. Serve with flatbread for dipping.

Nutrient Information: Approximate values per serving (excluding flatbread): Calories: 180, Protein: 9g, Fat: 7g, Carbohydrates: 23g, Fiber: 7g.

Mediterranean Breakfast Salad

Prep Time: 10 minutes

Ingredients:

- 1 cucumber, diced
- 2 tomatoes, diced
- 1/4 red onion, thinly sliced
- 1/4 cup crumbled feta cheese
- 2 tablespoons fresh herbs (e.g., oregano, mint)
- Lemon-oregano vinaigrette (2 parts olive oil, 1 part lemon juice, oregano, salt, and pepper)

Instructions:

1. In a large bowl, combine cucumber, tomatoes, and red onion.
2. Sprinkle feta cheese and fresh herbs over the vegetables.
3. Drizzle with the lemon-oregano vinaigrette and toss to combine.

Nutrient Information: Approximate values per serving: Calories: 120, Protein: 4g, Fat: 9g, Carbohydrates: 8g, Fiber: 2g.

Labneh and Za'atar Toast:

Prep Time: 5 minutes

Ingredients:

- 2 slices whole grain bread
- 1/2 cup labneh (strained yogurt)
- 1 teaspoon za'atar spice blend
- Olive oil for drizzling

Instructions:

1. Toast the bread until golden brown.
2. Spread labneh on the toasted bread slices.
3. Sprinkle with za'atar spice blend.
4. Drizzle with olive oil.

Nutrient Information: Approximate values per serving (2 slices): Calories: 250, Protein: 10g, Fat: 10g, Carbohydrates: 30g, Fiber: 5g.

Spanakopita

Prep Time: 45 minutes

Ingredients:

- 8 sheets phyllo dough

- 2 cups chopped spinach (frozen or fresh, well-drained)
- 1/2 cup crumbled feta cheese
- 1/4 cup chopped onions
- 2 tablespoons olive oil
- 1/2 teaspoon dried dill

Instructions:

1. Preheat the oven to 350°F (175°C).
2. In a pan, sauté onions in olive oil until translucent.
3. Add spinach, feta, and dill, and cook until combined.
4. Lay out one sheet of phyllo dough and brush with olive oil.
5. Place another sheet on top and repeat, creating 4 layers.
6. Cut the stacked phyllo sheets into squares.
7. Place a spoonful of the spinach mixture in the center of each square and fold into triangles.
8. Bake for about 25 minutes until golden and crispy.

Nutrient Information: Approximate values per serving (2 triangles): Calories: 150, Protein: 4g, Fat: 8g, Carbohydrates: 15g, Fiber: 2g.

Prep Time: 30 minutes

Ingredients:

- 1 pie crust (store-bought or homemade)
- 4 large eggs
- 1 cup milk
- 1/2 cup crumbled feta cheese
- 1/4 cup sliced olives
- 1/4 cup chopped artichoke hearts
- 2 tablespoons sun-dried tomatoes, chopped
- 1/4 teaspoon dried oregano

Instructions:

1. Preheat the oven to 375°F (190°C).
2. Beat the eggs and milk together in a large container.
3. Add feta, olives, artichoke hearts, sun-dried tomatoes, and oregano. Mix well.
4. Transfer the entire mixture into the pie crust.
5. Bake for 25-30 minutes or until the quiche is set and slightly golden.

Nutrient Information: Approximate values per serving (1/6 of the quiche): Calories: 300, Protein: 11g, Fat: 20g, Carbohydrates: 20g, Fiber: 2g.

Prep Time: 10 minutes

Ingredients:

- 2 slices whole grain bread, toasted
- 1 ripe avocado, sliced
- 1/4 cup crumbled feta cheese
- Drizzle of olive oil

Instructions:

1. Toast the bread until golden brown.
2. Top each slice with avocado slices.
3. Sprinkle with crumbled feta cheese.
4. Drizzle with olive oil.

Nutrient Information: Approximate values per serving (2 slices): Calories: 350, Protein: 9g, Fat: 20g, Carbohydrates: 32g, Fiber: 9g.

Mediterranean Chia Pudding

Prep Time: 10 minutes (plus chilling time)

Ingredients:

- 1/4 cup chia seeds
- 1 cup of almond milk (or any of your preferred choice of milk)
- 1 tablespoon honey
- 1/4 cup pomegranate seeds

- 2 tablespoons of finely chopped nuts, such as walnuts or almonds

Instructions:

1. In a jar, mix chia seeds and almond milk.
2. Stir in honey and combine well.
3. Cover the jar and refrigerate for at least 2 hours or overnight.
4. Before serving, top with pomegranate seeds and chopped nuts.

Nutrient Information: Approximate values per serving: Calories: 250, Protein: 6g, Fat: 15g, Carbohydrates: 25g, Fiber: 10g.

LUNCH

Greek Salad

Prep Time: 15 minutes

Ingredients:

- 2 large tomatoes, diced
- 1 cucumber, diced
- 1/2 red onion, thinly sliced
- 1/2 cup Kalamata olives, pitted
- 1/2 cup crumbled feta cheese
- Fresh oregano leaves

- Lemon-oregano dressing (2 parts olive oil, 1 part lemon juice, oregano, salt, and pepper)

Instructions:

1. In a large bowl, combine tomatoes, cucumbers, red onion, and olives.
2. Sprinkle crumbled feta over the top.
3. Garnish with fresh oregano leaves.
4. Drizzle with lemon-oregano dressing and toss to combine.

Nutrient Information: Approximate values per serving: Calories: 250, Protein: 7g, Fat: 20g, Carbohydrates: 12g, Fiber: 4g.

Mediterranean Falafel Wrap

Prep Time: 30 minutes

Ingredients:

- 4 falafel patties (store-bought or homemade)
- 4 whole wheat pita bread
- Toppings (e.g., lettuce, tomatoes, cucumbers, red onion)
- Tahini sauce

Instructions:

1. Heat the falafel patties according to package instructions or as per your recipe.
2. Warm the pita bread.
3. Place falafel in the pita and add your choice of toppings.
4. Drizzle with tahini sauce.
5. Wrap and serve.

Nutrient Information: Approximate values per serving: Calories: 350, Protein: 10g, Fat: 8g, Carbohydrates: 55g, Fiber: 8g.

Moussaka

Prep Time: 1 hour

Ingredients:

- 2 eggplants, sliced and grilled
- 1 lb ground meat (e.g., beef or lamb)
- 1 onion, chopped
- 3 cloves garlic, minced
- 1 can (14 oz) crushed tomatoes
- 1/2 cup red wine (optional)
- 1/2 teaspoon ground cinnamon
- 1/4 teaspoon ground nutmeg
- Salt and pepper to taste
- Bechamel sauce (butter, flour, milk, and nutmeg)

Instructions:

1. Grill eggplant slices until tender.
2. In a separate pan, brown the meat, onions, and garlic.
3. Stir in crushed tomatoes, wine, and spices. Simmer.
4. Layer a baking dish with eggplant, meat sauce, and bechamel.
5. Repeat layers and bake at 350°F (175°C) for 30-40 minutes.

Nutrient Information: Approximate values per serving (1/6 of the dish): Calories: 400, Protein: 15g, Fat: 18g, Carbohydrates: 30g, Fiber: 6g.

Tabbouleh Salad

Prep Time: 20 minutes

Ingredients:

- 1 cup of already cooked bulgur wheat (cooled)
- 1 cucumber, diced
- 2 tomatoes, diced
- 1/4 cup fresh parsley, chopped
- 1/4 cup fresh mint, chopped
- 1/4 cup red onion, finely chopped
- Lemon-olive oil dressing (2 parts olive oil, 1 part lemon juice, salt, and pepper)

Instructions:

1. In a large bowl, combine cooked bulgur, cucumber, tomatoes, parsley, mint, and red onion.
2. Drizzle with lemon-olive oil dressing and toss to combine.

Nutrient Information: Approximate values per serving: Calories: 250, Protein: 6g, Fat: 5g, Carbohydrates: 45g, Fiber: 10g.

Lentil Soup

Prep Time: 30 minutes

Ingredients:

- 1 cup of washed and drained lentils, either brown or green
- 1 onion, chopped
- 2 carrots, diced
- 2 celery stalks, diced
- 3 cloves garlic, minced
- 6 cups vegetable or chicken broth
- 1 teaspoon ground cumin
- Salt and pepper to taste

Instructions:

1. Fry the celery, carrots, and onions in a big-sized skillet until they are tender.
2. Add garlic and cumin and cook for another minute.

3. Stir in lentils and broth. Once it reaches a boil, lower the heat and simmer for approximately half an hour.
4. To your taste, add salt and pepper for seasoning.

Nutrient Information: Approximate values per serving (1/6 of the recipe): Calories: 250, Protein: 15g, Fat: 1g, Carbohydrates: 45g, Fiber: 12g.

Turkish Kebabs

Prep Time: 30 minutes (plus marinating time)

Ingredients:

- 1 lb boneless chicken, lamb, or beef, cut into cubes
- Marinade (olive oil, garlic, lemon juice, paprika, cumin, and oregano)
- Skewers
- chopped veggies, such as tomatoes, onions, and bell peppers

Instructions:

1. In a container, combine and mix the marinade ingredients.
2. Marinate the meat a minimum of half an hour.
3. Thread meat and vegetables onto skewers.
4. Grill or broil until cooked to your desired doneness.

Nutrient Information: Approximate values per serving: Calories: 250, Protein: 25g, Fat: 15g, Carbohydrates: 5g, Fiber: 1g.

Prep Time: 1 hour

Ingredients:

- Grape leaves (canned or fresh, blanched)
- Filling (rice, ground meat, onions, dill, mint, lemon juice)

Instructions:

1. Prepare the filling by mixing rice, ground meat, onions, dill, mint, and lemon juice.
2. Place a grape leaf shiny side down and add a spoonful of the filling.
3. Fold the sides and roll up the leaf into a small package.
4. Arrange dolmas in a pot, seam side down.
5. Add water, lemon juice, and olive oil to cover.
6. Simmer for 30-40 minutes.

Nutrient Information: Approximate values per serving (4 dolmas): Calories: 200, Protein: 5g, Fat: 10g, Carbohydrates: 25g, Fiber: 4g.

Couscous Salad

Prep Time: 20 minutes

Ingredients:

- 1 cup couscous, cooked and cooled

- An array of roasted vegetables, such as bell peppers, zucchini, and eggplant
- 1 tin (15 ounces) of chickpeas that is washed and have its water drained.
- Lemon-tahini dressing (tahini, lemon juice, garlic, water, salt, and pepper)

Instructions:

1. In a large bowl, combine couscous, roasted vegetables, and chickpeas.
2. Drizzle with lemon-tahini dressing and toss to combine.

Nutrient Information: Approximate values per serving: Calories: 350, Protein: 10g, Fat: 15g, Carbohydrates: 50g, Fiber: 8g.

Mediterranean Tuna Salad

Prep Time: 15 minutes

Ingredients:

- 2 drained 5-ounce cans of tuna in olive oil
- 1 cucumber, diced
- 1 cup cherry tomatoes, halved
- 1/4 cup of cut and pitted Kalamata olives
- 1/4 cup red onion, finely chopped
- 1/4 cup fresh parsley, chopped
- Feta cheese, crumbled

- Lemon-oregano vinaigrette (2 parts olive oil, 1 part lemon juice, oregano, salt, and pepper)

Instructions:

1. In a large bowl, combine tuna, cucumber, cherry tomatoes, Kalamata olives, red onion, and fresh parsley.
2. Top with crumbled feta cheese.
3. Drizzle with lemon-oregano vinaigrette and toss to combine.

Nutrient Information: Approximate values per serving: Calories: 300, Protein: 25g, Fat: 16g, Carbohydrates: 10g, Fiber: 2g.

Panzanella

Prep Time: 20 minutes

Ingredients:

- 4 cups stale Italian bread, cubed
- 2 cups cherry tomatoes, halved
- 1 cucumber, sliced
- 1/2 red onion, thinly sliced
- 1/4 cup fresh basil leaves, torn
- 1/4 cup fresh mozzarella, cubed (optional)
- Lemon-olive oil dressing (2 parts olive oil, 1 part lemon juice, garlic, salt, and pepper)

Instructions:

1. In a large bowl, combine stale bread, cherry tomatoes, cucumber, red onion, fresh basil, and mozzarella (if using).
2. Drizzle with lemon-olive oil dressing and toss to combine.
3. Let the salad sit for about 30 minutes to allow the flavors to meld.

Nutrient Information: Approximate values per serving: Calories: 250, Protein: 6g, Fat: 10g, Carbohydrates: 35g, Fiber: 4g.

DINNER

Grilled Lemon Herb Chicken

Prep Time: 30 minutes (plus marinating time)

Ingredients:

- 4 boneless, skinless chicken breasts
- Marinade (olive oil, lemon juice, garlic, herbs like rosemary and thyme)

Instructions:

1. Combine and mix together the marinade ingredients in a container.
2. Marinate the chicken for at least 30 minutes.

3. Grill the chicken until cooked through and juices run clear.

Nutrient Information: Approximate values per serving: Calories: 250, Protein: 30g, Fat: 12g, Carbohydrates: 3g, Fiber: 1g.

Ratatouille

Prep Time: 1 hour

Ingredients:

- 1 eggplant, cubed
- 2 zucchinis, cubed
- 1 red bell pepper, diced
- 1 onion, chopped
- 2 cloves garlic, minced
- 1 can (14 oz) crushed tomatoes
- Herbs (e.g., thyme, basil)

Instructions:

1. In a large pot, sauté onions and garlic until softened.
2. Add eggplant, zucchinis, and bell pepper. Cook until they start to soften.
3. Stir in crushed tomatoes and herbs. Simmer until vegetables are tender.

Nutrient Information: Approximate values per serving: Calories: 150, Protein: 3g, Fat: 1g, Carbohydrates: 35g, Fiber: 10g.

Prep Time: 45 minutes

Ingredients:

- 1 cup Arborio or Bomba rice
- 1/2 lb mixed seafood (e.g., shrimp, mussels, squid)
- 1/2 lb chicken or rabbit (optional)
- Saffron threads, soaked in warm water
- Vegetables (e.g., bell peppers, peas)
- Paprika, garlic, and onion
- Chicken broth

Instructions:

1. In a paella pan, sauté onion and garlic until translucent.
2. Add rice and saffron, stirring to coat.
3. Add chicken or rabbit (if using) and cook until browned.
4. Stir in paprika and vegetables.
5. Add seafood and enough chicken broth to cover the rice.
6. Simmer until the rice is cooked and the liquid is absorbed.

Nutrient Information: Approximate values per serving: Calories: 350, Protein: 20g, Fat: 10g, Carbohydrates: 40g, Fiber: 3g.

Prep Time: 1 hour

Ingredients:

- 4 bell peppers, halved and seeded
- Filling (ground meat, rice, tomatoes, herbs)

Instructions:

1. Prepare the filling by mixing ground meat, rice, diced tomatoes, and herbs.
2. Fill the bell pepper halves with the mixture.
3. Place in a baking dish, cover with foil, and bake at 375°F (190°C) for 40-50 minutes.

Nutrient Information: Approximate values per serving (1 stuffed pepper half): Calories: 200, Protein: 10g, Fat: 5g, Carbohydrates: 30g, Fiber: 4g.

Mediterranean Baked Salmon

Prep Time: 25 minutes

Ingredients:

- 4 salmon fillets
- Marinade (olive oil, lemon juice, garlic, herbs like dill and oregano)
- Sliced lemons and olives for garnish

Instructions:

1. In a container, combine together the marinade ingredients.
2. Marinate the salmon for about 15 minutes.
3. Preheat the oven to 375°F (190°C).
4. Place salmon fillets in a baking dish, pour the marinade over them, and garnish with lemon slices and olives.
5. Bake the salmon for approximately 15 to 20 minutes, or until it cracks easily.

Nutrient Information: Approximate values per serving: Calories: 350, Protein: 30g, Fat: 20g, Carbohydrates: 2g, Fiber: 0g.

Shrimp Scampi

Prep Time: 20 minutes

Ingredients:

- 1 lb large shrimp, peeled and deveined
- Linguine pasta
- Garlic, butter, and white wine
- flakes of Red pepper , parsley, and juice of lemon

Instructions:

1. Cook linguine according to package instructions.

2. Use butter to Fry garlic in a pan until it becomes fragrant.
3. Add shrimp and cook until pink.
4. Stir in white wine, lemon juice, and red pepper flakes.
5. Toss with cooked linguine and garnish with parsley.

Nutrient Information: Approximate values per serving: Calories: 350, Protein: 25g, Fat: 12g, Carbohydrates: 35g, Fiber: 2g.

Mediterranean Vegetable Stew

Prep Time: 1 hour

Ingredients:

- Assorted vegetables (e.g., eggplant, zucchini, bell peppers, tomatoes)
- Olive oil, garlic, onions, and herbs

Instructions:

1. In a large pot, sauté onions and garlic until softened.
2. Add a variety of vegetables and herbs.
3. Simmer until the vegetables are tender.

Nutrient Information: Approximate values per serving: Calories: 150, Protein: 2g, Fat: 7g, Carbohydrates: 20g, Fiber: 7g.

Prep Time: 30 minutes

Ingredients:

- 4 sea bass fillets
- Marinade (olive oil, lemon juice, garlic, herbs like thyme and rosemary)
- Sliced lemons and fresh herbs for garnish

Instructions:

1. In a container, combine together the marinade ingredients.
2. Marinate the sea bass for about 15 minutes.
3. Preheat the oven to 375°F (190°C).
4. Place sea bass fillets in a baking dish, pour the marinade over them, and garnish with lemon slices and fresh herbs.
5. Bake for 15-20 minutes or until the sea bass is cooked through and flakes easily.

Nutrient Information: Approximate values per serving: Calories: 300, Protein: 30g, Fat: 15g, Carbohydrates: 2g, Fiber: 0g.

Mediterranean Grilled Vegetable Platter

Prep Time: 20 minutes

Ingredients:

- A variety of veggies, including cherry tomatoes, bell peppers, zucchini, and eggplant
- Olive oil, garlic, and fresh herbs

Instructions:

1. Toss vegetables in olive oil, garlic, and fresh herbs.
2. Grill the vegetables until tender and slightly charred.
3. Arrange on a platter and serve with a dipping sauce like tzatziki.

Nutrient Information: Approximate values per serving: Calories: 150, Protein: 2g, Fat: 10g, Carbohydrates: 15g, Fiber: 5g.

SNACKS

Hummus with Veggies

Prep Time: 10 minutes

Ingredients:

- Hummus (store-bought or homemade)

- Assorted vegetables (e.g., baby carrots, cucumber, cherry tomatoes, bell pepper strips)

Instructions:

1. Arrange a selection of fresh vegetables on a platter.
2. Serve with a bowl of hummus for dipping.

Nutrient Information: Approximate values per serving (2 tablespoons hummus with veggies): Calories: 100, Protein: 3g, Fat: 6g, Carbohydrates: 10g, Fiber: 3g.

Greek Yogurt with Honey and Nuts

Prep Time: 5 minutes

Ingredients:

- Greek yogurt
- Honey
- Mixed nuts (e.g., almonds, walnuts, and pistachios)

Instructions:

1. Spoon Greek yogurt into a bowl.
2. Drizzle with honey.
3. Sprinkle with mixed nuts for added crunch and flavor.

Nutrient Information: Approximate values per serving: Calories: 200, Protein: 10g, Fat: 12g, Carbohydrates: 15g, Fiber: 2g.

Prep Time: 10 minutes

Ingredients:

- Assorted olives (e.g., Kalamata, green, and stuffed)
- Variety of cheeses (e.g., feta, halloumi, and goat cheese)
- Olive oil and herbs for drizzling

Instructions:

1. Arrange olives and cheese on a platter.
2. Drizzle with olive oil and sprinkle with herbs for added flavor.

Nutrient Information: Approximate values per serving: Calories: 250, Protein: 10g, Fat: 20g, Carbohydrates: 2g, Fiber: 1g.

Mediterranean Cucumber Cups

Prep Time: 15 minutes

Ingredients:

- Mini cucumbers
- Tzatziki sauce
- Cherry tomatoes and fresh dill for garnish

Instructions:

1. Slice the mini cucumbers into rounds.
2. Hollow out the centers to create "cups."

3. Fill each cucumber cup with tzatziki sauce.

4. Garnish with a cherry tomato slice and a sprig of fresh dill.

Nutrient Information: Approximate values per serving (2 cucumber cups): Calories: 50, Protein: 2g, Fat: 2g, Carbohydrates: 5g, Fiber: 1g.

Mediterranean Sardine Toast

Prep Time: 10 minutes

Ingredients:

- Whole grain bread, toasted
- Canned sardines in olive oil
- Sliced lemon, capers, and fresh herbs (e.g., parsley)

Instructions:

1. Top toasted bread with sardines, a slice of lemon, capers, and fresh herbs.

2. Serve as an open-faced sandwich.

Nutrient Information: Approximate values per serving (1 sardine toast): Calories: 150, Protein: 10g, Fat: 8g, Carbohydrates: 10g, Fiber: 2g.

Mediterranean Feta and Watermelon Bites

Prep Time: 15 minutes

Ingredients:

- Feta cheese, cut into cubes
- Watermelon, cut into cubes
- Fresh mint leaves
- Balsamic glaze (optional)

Instructions:

1. Skewer a cube of feta, a cube of watermelon, and a fresh mint leaf on a toothpick.
2. Drizzle with balsamic glaze if desired.

Nutrient Information: Approximate values per serving (2 bites): Calories: 50, Protein: 2g, Fat: 2g, Carbohydrates: 6g, Fiber: 1g.

Stuffed Dates with Almonds

Prep Time: 10 minutes

Ingredients:

- Medjool dates, pitted
- Whole almonds

Instructions:

1. Carefully slit each date and remove the pit.
2. Stuff an entire almond inside each date.

Nutrient Information: Approximate values per serving (2 stuffed dates): Calories: 80, Protein: 2g, Fat: 1g, Carbohydrates: 18g, Fiber: 2g.

Mediterranean Feta and Watermelon Bites

Prep Time: 15 minutes

Ingredients:

- Feta cheese, cut into cubes
- Watermelon, cut into cubes
- Fresh mint leaves
- Balsamic glaze (optional)

Instructions:

1. Skewer a cube of feta, a cube of watermelon, and a fresh mint leaf on a toothpick.
2. Drizzle with balsamic glaze if desired.

Nutrient Information: Approximate values per serving (2 bites): Calories: 50, Protein: 2g, Fat: 2g, Carbohydrates: 6g, Fiber: 1g.

Baba Ghanoush

Prep Time: 15 minutes

Ingredients:

- 2 large eggplants

- 3 cloves of garlic, minced
- 2 tablespoons of tahini
- 2 tablespoons of fresh lemon juice
- 2 tablespoons of ultra (extra) virgin olive oil
- 1/2 teaspoon of ground cumin
- Salt and black pepper to taste
- As a garnish, add some fresh parsley and a little olive oil.
- Pita bread, sliced vegetables, or pita chips for serving

Instructions:

1. Preheat your oven to 400°F (200°C).
2. Prick the eggplants with a fork in several places and place them on a baking sheet. Roast them in the preheated oven for about 30-35 minutes, or until the eggplants are soft and the skin is charred.
3. Remove the eggplants from the oven and let them cool for a few minutes.
4. Peel the skin from the eggplants and place the flesh in a bowl.
5. Mash the eggplant flesh with a fork or potato masher.
6. Add minced garlic, tahini, fresh lemon juice, extra virgin olive oil, ground cumin, salt, and black pepper to the mashed eggplant. Mix well to combine.
7. Transfer the baba ghanoush to a serving bowl, garnish with fresh parsley and a drizzle of olive oil.

8. Serve with pita bread, sliced vegetables, or pita chips for dipping.

Nutrient Information: (per serving) Calories: 67 kcal, Carbohydrates: 4.9g, Sugars: 1.45g, Protein: 0.95g, Fat: 5g, Saturated Fat: 0.7g, Fiber: 2.45g

Fried Calamari

Prep Time: 15 minutes

Ingredients:

- 1 pound of fresh calamari rings and tentacles
- 1 cup of all-purpose flour
- 1 teaspoon of paprika
- Salt and black pepper to taste
- Vegetable oil for frying
- Lemon wedges for serving

Instructions:

1. In a mixing bowl, combine the all-purpose flour, paprika, salt, and black pepper.
2. Heat vegetable oil in a deep frying pan or pot to 350°F (175°C).
3. Dredge the fresh calamari rings and tentacles in the seasoned flour mixture, ensuring they are coated evenly.
4. Carefully lower the coated calamari into the hot oil and fry for about 2-3 minutes, or until they are golden and crispy.

5. Remove the fried calamari from the oil and place them on a plate lined with paper towels to drain any excess oil.

6. Serve the crispy fried calamari with lemon wedges for squeezing over the top.

Nutrient Information (per 100g, without sauce): Calories: 200 kcal, Carbohydrates: 14g, Sugars: 1.3g, Protein: 17g, Fat: 8g, Saturated Fat: 0.9g, Fiber: 0.7g

Halloumi Cheese

Prep Time: 10 minutes

Ingredients:

- 8 slices of halloumi cheese (about 1/4 inch thick)
- 2 tablespoons of olive oil
- 1 lemon, cut into wedges
- Fresh mint leaves for garnish (optional)

Instructions:

1. Heat up a grill or grill pan over a moderate-high flame.
2. Brush the halloumi cheese slices with olive oil.
3. Grill the halloumi slices for about 2-3 minutes per side, or until they have grill marks and are slightly softened.
4. Arrange the grilled halloumi on a serving platter.
5. Use fresh mint leaves to garnish as preffered.

6. Serve with lemon wedges for squeezing over the cheese.

Nutrient Information (per serving): Calories: 160 kcal, Carbohydrates: 1.1g, Sugars: 0.55g, Protein: 10.5g, Fat: 12.5g, Saturated Fat: 8g, Sodium: 824mg

Loukoumades

Prep Time: 20 minutes

Ingredients:

- 1 cup of all-purpose flour
- 1 teaspoon of sugar
- 1/2 teaspoon of salt
- 1 packet which is about of 2 1/4 teaspoons of active dry yeast
- 1 cup of warm water
- Vegetable oil for frying
- Honey for drizzling
- Chopped nuts (usually walnuts or pistachios) for garnish (optional)

Instructions:

1. In a bowl, combine the all-purpose flour, sugar, and salt.
2. In a different container, Mix the yeast with a little warm water. Allow it to settle for five to ten minutes, or until foamy.

3. Pour the yeast mixture into the dry ingredients and mix to form a smooth batter. Cover the bowl and let it rest for about an hour, allowing it to rise.
4. Heat vegetable oil in a deep frying pan or pot to 350°F (175°C).
5. Drop spoonfuls of the batter into the hot oil and fry until they are golden brown and crispy, which takes about 2-3 minutes.
6. Remove the loukoumades from the oil and drain on paper towels.
7. Drizzle honey over the loukoumades and garnish with chopped nuts if desired.
8. Serve these sweet and fluffy loukoumades while they're still warm.

Nutrient Information (per serving): Calories: 160 kcal, Carbohydrates: 33g, Sugars: 10g, Protein: 3g, Fat: 2.5g, Saturated Fat: 0.35g, Fiber: 0.5g

Baklava

Prep Time: 45 minutes

Ingredients:

- 1 packet (16 oz.) of defrosted phyllo dough
- 2 cups of mixed nuts (walnuts, pistachios, or almonds), finely chopped
- 1 cup of unsalted butter, melted
- 1 teaspoon of ground cinnamon
- 1 cup of granulated sugar
- 1/2 cup of water
- 1/2 cup of honey
- 1 teaspoon of vanilla extract

Instructions:

1. Preheat your oven to 350°F (175°C).
2. In a bowl, combine the finely chopped nuts with ground cinnamon.
3. Brush a baking dish with melted butter and place one sheet of phyllo dough in the dish. Brush with more melted butter and continue layering and buttering each sheet until you've used half of the phyllo sheets.
4. Sprinkle the nut mixture evenly over the buttered phyllo layers.
5. Continue layering the remaining phyllo sheets, brushing each one with melted butter.
6. Use a sharp knife to cut the baklava into diamond or square shapes.
7. Bake in the preheated oven for about 45 minutes or until the baklava is golden brown and crisp.
8. While the baklava bakes, prepare the syrup. Put the granulated sugar, water, honey, and vanilla essence in a medium-sized saucepan. Allow it to boil, once it reaches a boil, lower the heat and simmer for ten minutes or so.
9. When the baklava is done, remove it from the oven and immediately pour the hot syrup over the hot baklava. Let it cool so the syrup may seep in.
10. Once the baklava has cooled, it's ready to be enjoyed.

Nutrient Information (per serving): Calories: 200 kcal, Carbohydrates: 36g, Sugars: 25g, Protein: 3.5g, Fat: 5g, Saturated Fat: 2g, Fiber: 0.7g

CONCLUSION

In closing, 'Mediterranean Diet Cookbook for Seniors 2024' is more than just a collection of recipes; it's a journey toward a healthier and more fulfilling life. We've explored the boundless flavors of the Mediterranean, and we've delved into the transformative potential of this remarkable diet.

The Mediterranean diet isn't just a meal plan; it's a way of life that nourishes both body and soul. As a senior, you hold the power to shape your health and vitality, and this book has been your faithful companion on that path. We've learned how to adapt the diet to your unique needs, embrace the benefits, and savor delectable, health-conscious meals.

Remember that your health and well-being are paramount, and the Mediterranean diet offers a roadmap to achieving your goals. By making mindful choices and savoring each bite, you're investing in a future of wellness and vitality.

But our journey doesn't end here. It's a lifelong adventure, and you have the tools and knowledge to keep moving forward. Embrace the flavors, cherish your health, and continue exploring the joys of the Mediterranean diet.

And as a token of our gratitude, we offer you a special bonus gift. Scan the QR code to access our meal planner, weight loss tracker, and blood sugar tracker. These tools are designed to support you on your path to better health.

If you've enjoyed your experience with this book and found it beneficial, we kindly ask for your feedback. Your review will help us continue to provide top-notch resources to seniors like you who are committed to their well-being. Your review and feedback are immensely valuable to us, and we thank you in advance for your time and input.

Thank you for coming on this adventure with us. We wish you the very best in your health and wellness journey.

Warm regards, Dr. Angela Cook

BONUS GIFT

MEAL PLANNER

MONDAY	BREAKFAST	
	DINNER	
TUESDAY	BREAKFAST	
	DINNER	
WEDNESDAY	BREAKFAST	
	DINNER	
THURSDAY	BREAKFAST	
	DINNER	
FRIDAY	BREAKFAST	
	DINNER	
SATURDAY	BREAKFAST	
	DINNER	
SUNDAY	BREAKFAST	
	DINNER	

NOTES

GROCERY LIST

WEIGHT LOSS TRACKER

WEEK: MONTH: YEAR:

DAY/DATE	WEIGHT	GAIN+	LOSS+	NOTES

BLOOD SUGAR LOG

WEEK: MONTH: YEAR:

DATE	TIME	LEVEL	NOTES

MEAL PLANNER

MONDAY	BREAKFAST	
	DINNER	
TUESDAY	BREAKFAST	
	DINNER	
WEDNESDAY	BREAKFAST	
	DINNER	
THURSDAY	BREAKFAST	
	DINNER	
FRIDAY	BREAKFAST	
	DINNER	
SATURDAY	BREAKFAST	
	DINNER	
SUNDAY	BREAKFAST	
	DINNER	

NOTES

GROCERY LIST

WEIGHT LOSS TRACKER

WEEK: **MONTH:**   **YEAR:**

DAY/DATE	WEIGHT	GAIN+	LOSS+	NOTES

BLOOD SUGAR LOG

WEEK: MONTH: YEAR:

DATE	TIME	LEVEL	NOTES

MEAL PLANNER

MONDAY	BREAKFAST	
	DINNER	
TUESDAY	BREAKFAST	
	DINNER	
WEDNESDAY	BREAKFAST	
	DINNER	
THURSDAY	BREAKFAST	
	DINNER	
FRIDAY	BREAKFAST	
	DINNER	
SATURDAY	BREAKFAST	
	DINNER	
SUNDAY	BREAKFAST	
	DINNER	

NOTES

GROCERY LIST

WEIGHT LOSS TRACKER

WEEK: MONTH: YEAR:

DAY/DATE	WEIGHT	GAIN+	LOSS+	NOTES

BLOOD SUGAR LOG

WEEK: MONTH: YEAR:

DATE	TIME	LEVEL	NOTES

MEAL PLANNER

MONDAY	BREAKFAST	
	DINNER	
TUESDAY	BREAKFAST	
	DINNER	
WEDNESDAY	BREAKFAST	
	DINNER	
THURSDAY	BREAKFAST	
	DINNER	
FRIDAY	BREAKFAST	
	DINNER	
SATURDAY	BREAKFAST	
	DINNER	
SUNDAY	BREAKFAST	
	DINNER	

NOTES

GROCERY LIST

WEIGHT LOSS TRACKER

WEEK: **MONTH:**   **YEAR:**

DAY/DATE	WEIGHT	GAIN+	LOSS+	NOTES

BLOOD SUGAR LOG

WEEK: MONTH: YEAR:

DATE	TIME	LEVEL	NOTES

MEAL PLANNER

MONDAY	BREAKFAST	
	DINNER	
TUESDAY	BREAKFAST	
	DINNER	
WEDNESDAY	BREAKFAST	
	DINNER	
THURSDAY	BREAKFAST	
	DINNER	
FRIDAY	BREAKFAST	
	DINNER	
SATURDAY	BREAKFAST	
	DINNER	
SUNDAY	BREAKFAST	
	DINNER	

NOTES

GROCERY LIST

WEIGHT LOSS TRACKER

WEEK: MONTH: YEAR:

DAY/DATE	WEIGHT	GAIN+	LOSS+	NOTES

BLOOD SUGAR LOG

WEEK: **MONTH:**   **YEAR:**

DATE	TIME	LEVEL	NOTES